So You Want To Be A Nurse

An innovative approach to success.

Dear Judy;

Thank you for your support. Please enjoy

Amira C.

Amira Clemens MSN RN

Table of Contents

Introduction 1

Acknowledgments 7

Welcome 11

What *Is* Nursing 17

Mastering the Textbook(s) 23

Studying.. 31

Believe In You 43

Make Friends... 51

Mentorship 59

Clinical.. 65

Networking Power 73

The Next Phase 83

Closing 91

Resources 97

Introduction

When I started nursing school, I learned a lot of things that were important to my success. I attended a workshop on how to do things like navigate the textbook, revise notes from class and how to study. Once I became an instructor, I learned things to have students do that would assist them with test preparation and success. This book is a collection of those things that came to be a significant and positive change in success for me and those seeking help from me. Another important element of this book is the importance of staying positive, believing in yourself and the influence energy has on the person. These are some things that are generally left out of moving through school, career choices and places of employment.

This book is a guide to help with achievement through nursing school. It is a collection of tips, tricks, and theories that have assisted many to a successful nursing career. Start to finish, it will help change your thinking about the nursing career and the good in it.

If you are considering nursing as a career choice, this is a nice tool that you can use to fill your time while you prepare for school to start or while you wait for your acceptance letter. It can also be used if you are stuck on something and need a reference.

This is a great gift for a new nursing student and a nice addition to other prep books like Nursing School Thrive Guide by Maureen Osuna. The rules of this book can also be translated to students in other careers. This has been written with nursing in mind but many of the chapters can be used as advice to a multitude of college and vocational students.

Lastly, this book is designed like a workbook. Extra pages are added to take notes or to complete the activity at the end of the subsequent chapters. So, mark it up as you see fit and keep it as a keepsake and reminder of things you wrote and therefore put into the universe.

Thank you for purchasing this book. If you did not purchase it (yet) I still would like to thank you for taking the time to consider this and reading the introduction.

Notes

Zavin Coles

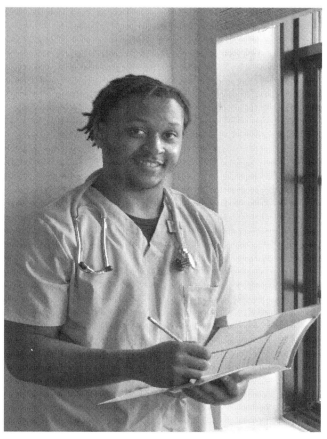

Notes

_____

_____

_____

_____

_____

_____

Acknowledgments

Mom

My mom is my biggest fan and supporter. She has no qualms about bringing me up in conversations that may have nothing to do with me or what I am doing. Almost everything I do in the community and in my career, is to make sure she is proud of me. This has been my goal since I was a child. If my mom is not happy with me or what I am doing, my life is not complete.

My children

Through some tough times in my life I looked to my children for balance. If they are doing well, all is well with me. Even as children, I went to them for advice. I got the green light from them to become a writer and for that I owe huge acknowledgement to them.

Zavin

Although Zavin is acknowledged above, I want to acknowledge him specifically. Whenever I needed a male prop for promo pictures, a volunteer, for anything, he is always up for it. I use him so much (pictured above as a nursing student) that his face is almost synonymous with my brand. He will also market things I am doing to his friends and on his social media page. I appreciate him so much!

Ameenah Diggins-Mahammad

Once I wrote this book I was stuck with the next steps. My friend Kenya recommended Ameenah to me and things were full speed ahead thereafter. Not only has she helped me with this book, but she has formulated some significant jewels of wisdom for all my entrepreneurial goals. I thank her for all that she has done and is continuing to do.

Jacqui and Kenya

When I needed some fresh faces to help with marketing and branding both Jacqui (my niece) and Kenya (good friend) stepped up without hesitation. Having people to agree to give their viewpoint, do a photoshoot and overall support is monumental. They are a blessing.

Dr. Waite

Dr. Waite is one of the major reasons that this book is completed. I had an idea, I created an outline, but I was not sure if I should move forward on this project. I met with her for lunch and although we talked about many things the idea for this book was included. She gave me full support and told me "that's a great idea." Because I hold her in high esteem as my mentor, I needed her blessing. I got it and the rest is history.

Friends and family

I have a long list of friends and family that I could list but the list would be a chapter long. My sisters, Shakera and Safiyah, my friends Sherrita and Denise have listened to me talk about this book for months. They evaluated pictures, paragraphs, and ideas from me on countless occasions. They have been my sideline of cheerleaders. I can't thank them enough.

To my other friends and family who provides immense support, this is for you. I love all of you and I am thankful that you are in my life. I am grateful to share this with you.

Notes

Chapter 1

WELCOME

"You have the power within yourself to make anything possible, you must diminish the doubt and ignite the self-belief."

-Leon Brown

Congratulatory Message

Let me first say congratulations on being accepted into nursing school. As you know from experience, getting accepted is not an easy process. You are about to embark on one of the scariest, most profound, confusing, and epic journeys of your life. I do not know why you chose nursing as a profession, but I am sure it was chosen with good reason and likely a good story behind it. In this book, I will share some of mine.

If you have not yet applied or been accepted, I would like to *still* congratulate you. Simply having an interest in nursing says a lot about you. Taking the time to read this book on how to navigate through nursing school prior to deciding to take that leap to apply or get accepted says even more.

Why this Book?

As a practicing nurse who also teaches, I see many nursing students and even active nurses who struggle with good study habits and how to structure routines that will lead to success. Also, the lack of understanding of the power of networking and relationship building. Considering the things that I did that made me a successful nursing student and, thereafter, that which I suggested for my students, I have compiled some of the information that I felt to be the most beneficial to anyone who is going to embark on this journey.

I was not unfamiliar with the healthcare field before going to nursing school. I was a Medical Assistant for more than six years before I went back to pursue a career in nursing. I had always known that health sciences were my niche and that I soared through all the things that got me through school and learning at work. So, going back to study nursing, specifically, made perfect sense.

In school, I had very good study habits from day one. The odd and uncanny things I did to remember things became some of the soundest advice I gave to my students once I became a professor. After years of giving advice and solutions on how to be a successful nursing student, and after years of mentoring new nurses, I decided to write this book as a blueprint to make the process a little smoother and to reduce some of the stress.

Pioneers of Nursing

As with many professions, there are people who enter the profession and leave a significant mark, be it an emotional change, invention, new practice, or an innovative way of doing things—there are many pioneers who came before you. Keep in mind that you also may become a pioneer of nursing.

The most notable pioneer who you should learn about is Florence Nightingale. It is her legacy that led you to this journey and maybe even this book. Learning about her and what she did for sick people (not just nurses) will give you some significant background information on how and why nursing is the amazing practice it is today.

Why it is the best profession ever

You likely know someone who is a nurse. In a ranking of professionals, nurses are among the most respected. But you may not know that nursing is one of the few careers to have HUNDREDS of options for the type of physical work that you can do. As a nurse, you should never be in a position that is unfulfilling, boring, or that you hate. There are just too many options.

Nurses care for people of all ages, from seconds to many years old. You can care for people in their most vulnerable and fragile to their happiest and most triumphant times. Some days you will leave school or work feeling like a superhero. There are not many professions that afford these emotions on a regular basis. This is what makes nurses special. You will truly feel like your job is one of the most important on the planet and you will not be wrong.

"The things you are passionate about are not random, they are your calling."

-Fabienne Fredrickson

Notes

_____

_____

_____

_____

_____

_____

_____

_____

_____

_____

_____

_____

_____

_____

_____

_____

_____

_____

_____

_____

_____

_____

_____

_____

_____

_____

_____

Chapter 2

WHAT *IS* NURSING

"Man's mind stretched to a new idea never goes back to its original dimensions."

-Oliver Wendell Holmes

What you may have thought

Of course, on the outside looking in, you may observe some things and draw a conclusion about what something or someone is. An auto mechanic looks like a person who knows their way around an engine. A businesswoman may appear to be well-kempt, poised, and have a lot of confidence. A school teacher may appear to be a very organized person. You get the picture. With a nurse, on the other hand, it is a little harder to tell. I personally believe that it is why nurses appear intriguing. As previously stated, nurses can work in a multitude of settings. That said, depending on where you see one and what they are doing, your assumption of a nurse will vary.

Some may think nurses are very smart people who learned how to do some complex medical procedures along with making sure people get medicine. Others might think nurses are people who can juggle multiple tasks at once and are important to maintaining a healthcare facility. And, on the dark side, some think nurses are glorified "butt wipers." The latter is not necessarily untrue.

What it is

Nursing is a science. Your degree or certificate, once you are done, will be in health science. Science, in its simplest explanation, is learning about things as they are broken down into their smallest part, assessing what they are and how all the small parts work together to complete the whole. In nursing, the information is broken down to understand people, their identity, and what they identify as. A mother, father, child, brother, sister, doctor, lawyer, pet owner, etc. Figuring how a disorder, injury, or disease is affecting that identity and how we as health care providers can get them back as close to that identity as possible.

It is a new language that you signed up to learn. Your first clinical day (in the hospital setting), listening in on the nurse-to-nurse reports, will be the best observation of this. You most certainly will not know what the nurses are talking about unless you are lucky enough to have considerate nurses who know that you are listening in and so speak in lay terms. But I am doubtful because this would make report longer and they will likely assume you understand. Don't stress. Just write it all down as best as you can and have your instructor translate it for you. "What is NPO, I's & O's, CBC's?" "I already know what a BM is." Over time, through reading, classroom lectures and continued clinical days, you will learn the language.

What you will soon learn

It is important. It is amazing. It is epic. You will come home with stories to tell for many years to come. Starting in nursing school, remember the excitement you have now, before beginning your career, and always remember it. Do not let go of the magic and you will love what you do indefinitely.

Nursing is one of those professions in which you must have a love for people and a desire to help those in need. It is true that some people come into nursing for the money because the jobs are plentiful. However, this cannot and must not be your drive to be in this profession. You will suffer. Your colleagues will suffer. Those you serve will suffer. It is not worth all the levels of misery that will ensue. It is not one of those things where it is the *norm* to be miserable simply because one has bills to pay. When it comes to doing something on a regular basis, happiness must be a part of that equation. Life is way too short and precious not to work towards being happy, as well as prosperous.

If you understand that this is not just a job but a thankless mission to serve, you will love it. It is also one of the few professions where you can do hundreds of different things as your *position*. That said, there is no reason to be unhappy. Do not believe that it is frowned upon to switch jobs or to not build a long work history. The only caveat is to be sure that you are building experience along the way. Once you have some experience under your belt, you can sell yourself from a learned perspective. You will know, from paying attention to those you meet and the things you learn, where you want to be in the future.

Try it

Most professions have a "process" through which skilled tasks are completed. Here is an activity to prepare you for the process you will use in your program:

Find someone you know who trusts you and will open up (you can also use yourself). Ask if they have a current or long-term injury, disorder, or illness. Answer the following questions…

1. What is it called?
2. What is it doing to the person's (or your) body?
3. What symptoms does it cause?
4. What, if any, medications are taken for it?
5. What do the healthcare workers (specifically nurses) do to help?

If you have completed this activity, you have completed a simplified version of the Nursing Process. Understanding and doing this for every issue discussed will help you understand how nurses care for people.

Notes

_____

_____

_____

_____

_____

_____

_____

_____

_____

_____

_____

_____

_____

_____

_____

_____

_____

_____

_____

_____

_____

_____

_____

_____

_____

Chapter 3

MASTERING THE TEXTBOOK(S)

"Books may be irrelevant until its relevance, importance, and purpose is discovered through reading."

-Ernest Agyemang Yeboah

Get them

Whether you are coming into nursing as a traditional student, non-traditional, or in a fast track from another degree, the topic always comes up. "Should I get the books?" Some will even ask the instructor if they need them. Please refrain from asking that.

Not getting the books for a specified class is a recipe for disaster. I am fully aware that there are many courses that you can do this. Nursing is NOT one of them. It is a huge gamble. Are there people who survive nursing school on PowerPoints and Google? Yes! But the chances of you succeeding using only these resources is statistically too small, so you shouldn't even try it. Even if you only open a book once in any given class, it is worth it! The textbooks will save your career as a student.

Consider the type of resources you prefer. Some like a physical book. Others like electronic versions. Ask if your preferred type is available. Also, be sure to choose the most practical. Sometimes the version you do not like will be the cheapest. Find a sensible medium when it comes to this. If you cannot afford either, most schools have a reserve copy of the required textbooks in the school's library. It may be an inconvenience to go there to use it, but it is another activity that will be worth it in the end. If you must use the reserved copy, make the trip worth it. Plan to stay and study as much as you can while you are there.

Textbooks are tools. Not getting them is equivalent to a handyman showing up at someone's house to do work and asking the customer if they have a hammer—one of the basic tools to do most jobs. You need them to complete the information that is introduced in the class. You need them as a point of reference. You need them to study. Get them!

Use them

You can most certainly *not* learn everything you will need to know and be responsible for in class. You need textbooks as much as a spelling bee contestant needs a dictionary. And you must set aside time to use them.

- Make appointments to go over the information in your texts.
- Put it on a calendar and respect it as much as you would your class schedule.
- Schedule everything! Class, reading, studying, eating, bathing, cleaning, laundry… I am only half kidding.

You must remain in control while in nursing school. Once you are done with the program you can be relaxed with your time, but in nursing school developing rituals and a routine is paramount. One small issue can make things spiral out of control very easily. This is not to say that trying to maintain control will keep things from happening, but it will keep everything from seeming like it will fall apart. A sense of control is important in nursing school.

When you get your syllabi for each class, take some time to review the topics that will be covered each week.

- With your schedule and the topic reading list, make an outline on a Word document or sheet of paper. Do this every week.
- Make note of the specifics that will be covered.
- Make your outline match the way the information is covered in the text.
- Create headings, subheadings, and bullet points.
- Leave space in your outline to take notes in class.
- After class, in the time slot you scheduled, complete the information that you learned in class by using information from the textbook.

I have included a sample outline for you to view or use as you see fit. Keep in mind that you may need to adjust my sample.

Pro-tip: research has shown that the actual act of writing things down by hand, not typing on a computer, helps solidify the intended knowledge and memory of a learning event. You use more neurosynapses writing things than you do typing. Just saying!

Master them

Using the method of accumulating the information above (outlines, lecture emphasis, and textbook inclusion) you will have the most impeccable documents. This will become your best study tool when exams and quizzes are coming up. You won't have to spend time with the text in preparation because you will have done that already and have all the information you need. More information on preparing for quizzes and exams are in another chapter.

Completing Anatomy and Physiology will help you with a basic understanding of the body and how all the systems work together. If it has been a while since you have taken it before being accepted into nursing school, go back to refresh your memory and understanding using your notes or an old textbook. Understanding the responsibility of each system will help you with what happens when a specific system is not doing its job. Once you feel like you are comfortable with your background knowledge of the body, have your body system to be discussed in class, review the specific diseases but only to learn the gist of them. In nursing, you will need to know what your responsibility is to the person with the disease being discussed. You should spend most of your time reviewing and learning the nursing/collaborative care of the issue. This means that you will spend most of your time getting the most understanding of that section of the chapter in your text. A lot of textbooks will provide you with an immense amount of information about a disease or disorder. It does not mean that you should spend a lot of time memorizing diseases. Remember that nurses treat the person, not the disease. The background information is there to make the information complete. Your use of the textbook should be on the nursing responsibility and critical thinking.

Another big activity involving the text is being sure that you take time to learn the terms. This is something a lot of nursing students neglect. As stated in a previous chapter, nursing is a language. You will not understand what you are being asked if you don't take the time to learn the terms. Some schools mandate taking a medical terminology course. I highly recommend this if it is an option for you prior to starting to nursing school. If it is not mandatory, you can go to your local library to get resources to learn how medical terminology works. It is not just about learning words and meanings; it is learning which root words, prefixes, and suffixes are used in health science. Learning how medical terminology works will allow you to dissect most all words in nursing school to learn their meanings.

If you know your terms, you know what is being talked about and what you are being asked. This includes class, clinical, and tests. Not knowing your terms can be like going to a foreign country and trying to get around without knowing how to ask questions or what you are being told.

You won't be sorry

If you were to able to speak to and compare the experiences of those who had a minimally stressful ride in nursing school to those who were stressed and barely got by (by the skin of their teeth), I am confident that the statistics would show that the structured and prepared student would report that their time was difficult but not out-of-control stressful. Please note that nursing school is difficult. No matter where you go to school do not believe that your "hell" is isolated to where you chose to go to school. I promise that taking time to prepare and use the tools available will make nursing school more bearable.

Sometimes, you will feel like you are being hit with more information than you can handle. There are going to be days when you go home feeling like your brain is vibrating with all the information you received that day. The one thing that you will have control over is navigating the text. Having a sense of control of at least one source of information will significantly help. Mastering the text will give you that. It will also provide a solid foundation for other information you encounter from other sources. You will feel less lost and you will not have to spend as much time looking up information as an afterthought.

Try it

To estimate the power in routines and habits you must formulate a structure and stick to it like your life depends on it. Set a schedule for yourself and treat it like it is from your employer. Here is a trial of this:

1. Get a calendar or calendar book.
2. Make a list of things you MUST accomplish and things you WANT to accomplish within the next week.
3. Prioritize the tasks.
4. Put the most difficult and intricate tasks at the top of the list.
5. Schedule each item within your calendar. Make sure you are as realistic as possible with your timeline to complete them. Set an intention to complete the difficult tasks first.
6. Complete each task by the date you set, NO MATTER WHAT.

If you take the time to complete this activity, then you will learn the significant sense of accomplishment afforded by staying on schedule, crossing items OFF your to-do list and being loyal to yourself. We often put the things we must do for ourselves last because we believe we must do things for others first. Family, work, friends, then ourselves. This has an impact on how we value ourselves, even if it is not apparent. Put yourself at the top of your priority list and this will begin to change.

Sample Outline

Topic

(System or Disease)

Definition

- What is it?
- Where is it?

Terms

- What are the specific terms (words) used when discussing this?

Etiology

- What is its significance?
- What is it doing?
- Why is it doing this?
- Where is it doing this?

Signs and Symptoms

- What will the person complain of?
- What changes will they see?
- What are the urgent symptoms?

Medication (Pharm)

- What medicine will be taken for this?

Collaboration

- What other health professionals will play a part in care?
- What will they do?
- What is their specialty?

Patient Teaching

- What is going on?
- How can we prevent things from getting worse?
- What do you need to report to the nurse or doctor?

Interventions

- What are the most important things I need to do?
- What is a good outcome?
- What should I do if things don't get better?

Notes

Chapter 4

STUDYING

"Tell me and I'll forget. Show me and I may remember. Involve me and I learn."

-Benjamin Franklin

Why

Some of the people who come to nursing may have very good study habits, others could potentially have never studied. Some are so fortunate to have never needed to. As previously stated, it is a gamble and not worth it. One of the most pivotal methods of success in nursing school is studying and making time to study. If you already have good study habits, then keep them. Do not reinvent the wheel. But if you find that your methods don't work for nursing, try my suggestions. If not mine, then someone else's that you feel will work. I would love to say that my method is the gold standard, but that would be untrue. Does my method work? Absolutely! Just not with everyone, every time. It is simply the concept of my method that is important. Get the info. Review it. Become familiar with it. Learn it. Trust it.

An important part of my study concepts is developing routines. There is power in routines. Our routines are what define us as a person. The things that we purposely do, every day, by deeply rooted routines, that we learned from our parents or upbringing, is what develops our character.

- A "morning person" gets up early every morning no matter what.
- An athlete works out every day.
- There are people who eat the same food for breakfast.

Their routines stay the same. It is who they are. However, routines are not set in stone. They are fluid. They can be changed and redeveloped. There are routines that you can develop in nursing school that are just for nursing school that define you as a nursing student. Once you complete the program, you can redefine yourself and routines as a new nurse. The persistence in maintaining routines help give strength and confidence, both of which are important characteristics to be successful.

The knowledge that you gather on specific topics begins in reviewing the lesson and in class with the lecture. The important thing to consider in studying is that it is a method of gathering information, processing it, and knowing it. For this to happen successfully and for you to solidify it, you must be PRESENT. What does this mean? It means that being in class, reading your textbook, structuring or reviewing your notes should all be done with your undivided attention. Your phone should be off or tucked away and silent. There should not be any background noise unless it is music with instruments only. If you use your computer in class, shut off all notifications. Give all learning activities your attention. Dividing your attention weakens the learning process. Multitasking is a myth! I am aware that this is difficult these days with cellphone addiction and the constant multiple stimuli we encounter all day. But it is very possible to focus your attention. Once you learn how to do it, embrace it and use it, it will become a part of your routine and your personality.

How

Using the information from chapter four will prepare you for studying. It is my position that studying starts on the first day of class. It is ongoing and not a specific event. If you use the method of taking notes that I suggested in chapter three, then you are already in study mode.

Once you have all the outlines that you created in preparation for the class, you have the basic tools to start studying. However, the method that I will suggest for using your notes is different than some of the study methods you may be used to. It will also save you from having to sacrifice a whole day, evening or even weekend to prepare. My suggestions are:

- Start day one (or week one if you are in a fast track program).
- Read the notes you made as soon after class as you have the time. It is best the same day or within 24 hours.
- Simply read them once. The only other suggestion outside of reading them is completing a thought and correct some spelling while your read.
- Read your notes every day. At least once.
- Each subsequent set of notes should be read backward.

- So, you will read:

  1. The notes from the current day.
  2. Next, read the notes from the previous day.
  3. Continue to read until you've read up to the notes you took on the very first day.

- Within a month's time, you will be completely familiar with the information.
- The information from day one or the furthest away from the test (usually the overview of the topic) will be solidified.

Let me break this down differently… if you have class on Monday, Tuesday, and Wednesday, for example, you will read/edit Monday's notes on Monday, on Tuesday you will read Tuesday's notes then read/edit notes from Monday, and on Wednesday you will read notes from Wednesday, then Tuesday and finally read/edit notes from Monday. You carry this on until the quiz or exam for the information or until you have confidence that you know the content.

The best explanation for the above method is that you are not looking at information from the beginning weeks after you've recorded it and you may not remember the points that were emphasized. It is not best practice to wait until a day or two before an exam to read your notes and the textbook. You will find it overwhelming and it can induce anxiety, then block learning from occurring.

The final thing you need to do to prepare for exams and quizzes is practice questions. There are a lot of nursing students who do not use this method. It is extremely important to test your own knowledge. You do this by utilizing practice questions. Test-taking strategies are part of learning and understanding nursing information. I promise you the type of questions you will encounter in nursing school are like no other test questions you have ever seen. A nursing student is setting themselves up to fail if they do not practice test taking. I use the analogy of a football team. A team cannot go play a game simply by watching plays on videos and listening to the coach explain them. They must get on the field and practice the game. The same goes for practice questions.

Go get a study guide that accompanies the textbook or a good NCLEX practice book. The best type of NCLEX book is one that has the body/disease systems categorized rather than one with randomized questions. Make time to work the practice questions in the same way you make time to study. Allot a specific amount of practice questions per topic as a goal for yourself every week. The number of questions you work should vary by your weaker versus stronger knowledge of a subject. You should also look at the reasoning for the correct and incorrect answers provided. This will help close the gap in understanding. Especially if you *guessed* the correct answer and only got it right by default. It will make a huge difference.

There are also apps you can get on your smartphone that can provide you with the option to solve practice questions. This is especially good for those who are on their devices a lot and use them during downtime. Like waiting for food, standing in line, or using the bathroom. I encourage you to use whatever you must, to reach your goals. However, I am a fan of the pen to paper, highlighting, and more active learning activities. The method is up to you. Just be sure you do it.

A bonus method that I find to be helpful with learning information is using Post-it® notes. There will be times that you will have to be familiar with number ranges, lab values, and unfamiliar terms that you find hard to remember. If you write it on a Post-it® note and put it somewhere you will encounter it throughout your day, then it will help you recall the information when you need to. Place them inside the jacket of a folder you use often, the bathroom or vanity mirror, a closet door, etc.

This is not good practice for a whole list of definitions because you may raise some concern by your friends and family as to why you have an entire wall with notes stuck to it. Only use it for those things that you feel are hard to remember because you can't relate it to something else. Once you learn it and feel confident that you will remember it, take the note down. Or take it down at the end of the course for which you needed it.

You must take the time to practice and solidify the information in your mind. Speaking of the athletes, it is not good practice to wait until right before a competition or meet to train. You will lack confidence and the odds of winning will be reduced to the same as a single coin toss. Therefore, studying is one of the most powerful tools for succeeding in nursing school. How you study is also important. If you repeat something every day it becomes part of your conscious and subconscious. Just as hearing your name gets your attention. You know your name. It has been repeated millions of times in your life. That part of the spoken language and your brain have connected you with instantly paying attention when you hear your name called. Having the ability to recall information cannot come from spending a short amount of time reviewing. And the information in nursing school cannot be memorized or crammed. You must have a clear understanding of the concepts, or, minimally, be familiar with them. That only comes with regular practice. Repetition works.

As a method of maintaining good mental health, you should give yourself a break from the information prior to an exam. It may not be necessary prior to a short quiz. This is more significant at times prior to a midterm or final exam. Give yourself some downtime. If you have stuck to your study schedule and have been doing well with your practice questions, you are ready. You have done what you needed to do. Trust your training and take a break. The night before your major exams, put all your books away, log off your computer, and take it easy. Have a good dinner with friends or family, take a walk, watch TV, take a bath, meditate… GET A GOOD NIGHT'S SLEEP. It is not necessary to keep the same momentum if you have been doing what you needed to do up to that point. In fact, studies show, that you decrease your chances of doing well if you don't have a cutoff and continue to look at the information all the way up to the exam time. You will likely see something you think you overlooked, not have the time to research it, and anxiety will kick in. You will question your knowledge of everything and potentially blank out due to the overwhelming anxiety. If you understand how the subconscious works, you will have faith that it will rise to the occasion.

Speaking of "the exam time," it is also a good idea to either walk into class right on time or wear some headphones while waiting for the exam to be administered. The chatter from your classmates can also be a distraction and another source of anxiety. It would be nice if everyone sat quietly, looking at their notes prior to an exam, but this just does not happen. Once the exam is over, leave. Do not hang out and discuss the exam afterward with ANYONE. If you are done for the day, go home. Have another relaxing evening. If you have class, find somewhere quiet or, once again, use those headphones and block out the aftermath chatter. What's done is done. There is no need to stress over the unknown. You will find that all that anxiety would have been a waste. Even if you did not do as well as you would have liked to, place it on your list of things to revise.

Revising

Once you have taken an exam or quiz, assess where your weaknesses are, be it a specific system or disease, or terms or test taking in general. Look at the areas for improvement so that your scores stay consistent if you did well or get better if there is a need to.

During this time, you may consider some mistakes you made. Maybe even a mistake in judgment. Like... changing an answer from correct to incorrect. A common mistake nursing students make. Here's my take on changing answers:

> "Your subconscious mind will tell you the correct answer before your conscious mind can talk you out of it. Therefore, never change your answer unless you are 100% sure you read the question wrong."

> -Unknown

Revising your plans and restructuring your focus based on the feedback from those questions you got wrong, mistakes you make in projects, or errors on papers builds resilience. Remember that you are a student. Students are learners. Some students forget the process of learning and what it means to be a student. *It means* that you don't know all the information. *It means* you are in the process to develop into the person that learning will give you. *It means* that it is normal to not get perfect grades. Perfect grades don't allow growth. This does not mean that getting 100% is bad. *It means* that once you get that perfect grade, you no longer feel the need to revisit any of that information contained in that assessment and you will not continue to grow. Of course, there are going to be things that you know and know well. That it is understood why you got a perfect score. But the important thing is that perfect scores should not be an expectation of a student and "lack-thereof" is not a reflection of the instructor.

Unusual Study Practices

When it comes to preparing for anything in life we tend to follow and prepare using methods that we learned from those who have an influence on us. We may learn from our mothers to clean and organize when company is coming. This is an example. We know that this is not something we have to do to have visitors, but it makes us feel better and allows the visit to be better. There are certain things we do that give us confidence even though they are not necessary, but the key thing here is confidence. So here is a list of things that I and others have done to prepare for exams. Some are backed by science and others are known to work with no plausible explanation.

1. Listen to classical music while studying. Have it playing at a low but audible level in the background. It helps the brain function better.
2. Drink water. Our body, including our brains, are mostly water. When we become dehydrated our body and brain do not function properly. Drinking water helps with increased alertness and increased mental function.
3. Chew gum or suck on hard candy of specific flavor while studying. Chew the same flavored gum or candy during the exam. The familiar flavor will help recall the information reviewed during studying in the same way a familiar scent brings back memories.
4. Wear something bright colored like orange or yellow. Or, have something orange or yellow within the visual field during the exam like a pen or pencil. Bright colors increase neurosynaptic function, so our brain activity is increased when it is needed.

5. Eat some chocolate (if you like it and are not allergic) during the exam. The sugar and caffeine will increase energy and brain function.

6. Organize your notes and textbook topics. Put them in order and make a recording of your own notes in a controlled setting. Listen to them every day until the exam on the topics. A lot of students like to record the professor in a lecture. This is good for reference, but this activity is different. You have the information you need to learn, and you are listening to it in your own voice. It is specific, organized, and free of the distractions and side conversations of the lecture recording. It is like telling yourself the information you need to know in a story. Hearing it in your own voice also has a significant impact on your subconscious mind.

7. Read your notes or schedule study time at night before bedtime. You remember the information that you take in before bedtime because there are fewer interactions with your subconscious mind. Therefore, information taken in before sleep is recalled more easily.

Notes

Chapter 5

BELIEVE IN YOU

"A man is literally what he thinks, his character being a complete sum of all his thoughts."

-James Allen; As A Man Thinketh

There is power in thoughts

People who are spiritually driven will understand this portion of the book. It may sound "woo woo" otherwise. But through some easy research on the subject, you will find how simple and powerful this concept is.

If you knew how influential thoughts were, you'd carefully choose them all day. Thoughts become things. Your current reality is generated by your thoughts. Let's evaluate this book if you will. Everything that you are reading at this moment was once my thoughts. Yet now you have this book in your possession. It is the *thing* I have created with my thoughts—an idea to write this book. Look around the room or space that you are currently in. Look at where you are sitting, any pictures on the walls, buildings, furniture, anything… All those items were created out of someone's thoughts. Things don't have to be tangible. They can also be an outcome. I thought I wanted to be an author. I wrote this book. I am an author. You thought you wanted to go to nursing school. You went through all the steps to get there. You are now (or potentially are) a nursing student. EVERYTHING begins with a thought; think positive!

"Our life is what our thoughts make it."

-Marcus Aurelius Antonius

Another powerful action is to write things down. Whether it be setting goals or personal reminders, writing things down sets them into motion. Having things in our minds, and not on paper, keeps them as an idea or wish. The act of writing things down takes it from a thought or an intangible thing to something real. Especially a goal. Goals are simply wishes if they are not written down. Writing ideas and goals down is a game changer and sets things to come to life. Therefore, daily and weekly goals can be one of the most significant habits that lead to success. Take some time every week to set intentions for the things you want to achieve for that week. It could be a small goal, like reading over notes, a page in your textbook, or sending an email. If it is important, write it down as an intended task to complete for the week. Over time, when you look back at the things you set to tackle, you will gain a sense of accomplishment when you see how much you have accomplished. So, no task is too small. Many small tasks will lead to big achievements.

We have so many thoughts and ideas every day and all day. If those thoughts are things you really want or need to accomplish, make it a point to write them down or type them out. With so many thoughts and ideas, it is nearly impossible to remember which of those tasks are important. Put it on paper. If it is time sensitive, put it on a calendar. Write it down. Take those thoughts, ideas, and timed tasks and set intentions. Write intentions for every month, every week, and every day. Whatever you do, write out your intentions. When you complete your tasks, cross them off. This is a tremendous means of achievement.

Goals are what drive us. It is what makes us get up out of bed every day.

- To go to school—we want to finish.
- To go to work—to get money.
- Meet with friends—to have fun.

Most of our daily actions are to complete goals. Writing out our intentions and completing them are purposeful goals that we create and complete as we cross them off. Accomplishing goals has an amazing effect on our sense of self and self-esteem.

"Setting goals is the first step in turning the invisible into the visible."

-Tony Robbins

Stay positive

Consider the power in thoughts and you will understand the power in staying positive. It is dangerous to allow negative emotions to lead you. Nursing school is stressful. Period! But if you adhere to the stressful persona, you will occasionally be defeated by your negative emotions. If you believe in the power of the universe, you understand that your life will reflect the energy you put out.

Energy is like karma. If you continue to put out negative energy, your life will feel and reflect negativity. Guess what? Just because you are going through something difficult does not give you the green light to be negative and identify with your stressors. Positivity, like happiness, is a choice. It also comes from within. Remaining positive does not mean that all your stress will automatically disappear. However, you will experience less of it and you will not allow it to lead you.

> "Keep your thoughts positive because your thoughts become your words. Keep your words positive because your words become your behavior. Keep your behavior positive because your behavior becomes your habits. Keep your habits positive because your habits become your values. Keep your values positive because your values become your destiny."

-Mahatma Gandhi

You must believe

To be successful, at anything, you must first believe you WILL be. You do not and should not leave things up to chance. Create what you want by believing it is possible.

If you took the time to study, prepare, and complete all the necessary tasks up to an evaluation, why would you believe that you will fail? Confidence should be radiating from you. This is exactly what confidence is. It is the *knowledge* that you did all you needed to do to get where you are. So why would you fail? You simply must believe. There is also power in belief. Believing in yourself significantly increases your chances of success. If you were able to talk to any performance athlete and ask them, what it is that makes them confident in their ability to win. I am sure it would be unanimous that it is the belief that they will win. If you want to be confident, you only need to believe.

Affirmations are statements we make to ourselves that support emotional encouragement. They are declarations that we make either out loud, to ourselves, or on paper—a method of programming your subconscious mind in a positive way. Whenever you feel stressed, take three deep breaths and say these affirmations out loud:

- I am confident.
- I am strong.
- I am powerful. This really works!

Another action of success is being grateful. Gratitude changes us from having a grim outlook on life and current situation, to have an extremely positive outlook. Once you learn to be thankful and pay attention to the things you should be thankful for, more things come your way. That is the way the universe works. It is not just negative things happening to "bad" people getting served their karma. The more you are appreciative, the more you will have a positive outlook, and more things to be appreciative of.

> "If you continually give, you will continually have."
>
> -Unknown (Fortune Cookie)

If you did not do well on a quiz or exam, if you got an unsatisfactory evaluation, or must redo an assignment but you are still in the program and have a chance to recover, look at the good. Be thankful that you still have a chance to succeed. Take the lesson in what you did wrong and how you can improve, and then work on new goals. Remember that educational programs are for you to learn and grow. It is normal to have room for improvement. It does not make you a bad student because you did not do well on one specific portion of a class or topic.

Try it

Gratitude can significantly change your perception of life. However, it takes time and effort to learn how to make time to be grateful. This is not to say that you are not thankful for the things you have. What I am saying is that a lot of us don't realize that we have way more things to be grateful for than we account for. We sometimes complain about what we don't *have* and those things we don't *like* way more than we take account of the abundance in our lives.

Get a sheet of paper or an old notebook, put the date on the top, and write out five things that you are grateful for. Do not simply make a list. Put a short explanation for why you are grateful for these items. This could be a list of people as well. Do this for a week. Do not let the list be shorter than five items. Do not repeat items for the subsequent days unless there is a different reason you are thankful for it. A list could include anything and look like this:

1. I am thankful for my brain that helps me think through complex problems.
2. I am thankful for my hands that I use all day to touch and pick up things including food that I put in my mouth.
3. I am thankful for my children who give me the drive to keep reaching my goals, so I can be a positive role model for them.

I would bet that your perception of life and the abundance you have would start to change. If you keep it up, you will change indefinitely.

Notes

Chapter 6

MAKE FRIENDS

"Try leaving a friendly trail of the little sparks of gratitude on your daily trips. You will be surprised how they will set small flames of friendship that will be rose beacons your next visit."

-Dale Carnegie; How to Win Friends and Influence People

Support

It is well and widely known that developing a system of support create positive outcomes. It is why programs like Weight Watchers are so popular and the participants have a higher level of success in comparison to those trying to lose weight alone. In nursing school, it is extremely important to make friends. It is also important for these friends to be made in the school you are currently in. No one else in your life will understand what you are going through during your time in nursing school as much as someone going through it along with you. Right next to you!

However, it is important for you to be careful who you choose to befriend. It is not necessary to study people or administer applications, but you want to be selective. You don't want to end up being in the company of someone who drains your energy or one who has an unhealthy emotional attachment. This can be counterproductive. Entering into a new venture can be scary. People who are afraid tend to latch on to others as a source of security. Especially those who appear confident or stoic. Be mindful that you must find people who can uplift you and that you have a supportive connection with.

Pay attention to those whose energy matches yours. Ones with whom you find it easy to talk to and who give you a sense of comfort when you are around them. Once I had some exams under my belt and it was known that I was doing well, certain people began to pay attention to me. Especially those who were struggling and were looking for someone on their level to latch on to. There was one student who wanted to study with me who taught me a lesson in being careful with whom you study. She asked to be a study partner, but what she ended up doing was looking to me for tutoring. I am sure that this was not purposeful, but it is what happened. She did not offer anything to me in the learning process. In fact, after studying with her, I got the lowest test score of my nursing school career. As bad as I felt for her struggles, I had to disconnect and be solo until I found someone with whom learning could be reciprocated.

It is also a method of survival to cut some people off. This may sound like it contradicts the previous suggestions. Hear me out. There will be people who you may have issues with prior to nursing school. You will have to avoid them. Your ability to tolerate them and their negative effects on you will decrease as they will not understand, help, or benefit your journey. You most certainly can reconnect with them after graduation, if you see fit. But do not feel guilty for putting them on the back burner to focus on yourself and your goals. This includes select family members as well. You will have the rest of your life to make it up to them.

As unfortunate as it is to state, it is a reality for some to experience strained relationships during this time. Why is this? I have my speculations, but I am not sure. I have heard it enough times NOT to ignore and omit it from this book. There are people who have significant others who try to intentionally sabotage their efforts to get a solid career by going to school. Of course, this is not isolated to nursing school, but nursing school is not exempt. It is enough for me to say to pay attention and be careful. It can cause expensive, emotional, and destructive damage—a fact that may not be known until you are well into the program. If you find this to be true for you, do not ignore it. Find help or solutions.

If you have supportive friends and family, you are truly fortunate. Embrace and thank them as often as possible. Sometimes major sacrifices go into going back to school. Not everyone will understand what this means. If you have people in your life who not only understand, but also supports this goal, you have an immeasurable blessing. Hold on to them for dear life!

There is a truthful statement and belief that we are the product of the five people we spend the most time with. If they are negative and unmotivated, you will find yourself negative and unmotivated by being in their company. If they are driven and inspired, you will absorb their energy and become the same. Knowing and understanding this means that you will start paying attention and becoming selective. Napoleon Hill stated in his book *Think and Grow Rich*, that many of the successful people in history had what is called a "Master Mind Group." This is a group of people who are dedicated to see a successful outcome and share common goals. The power in these groups is the synergy that develops and create outcomes that would be difficult and time-consuming if attempted by a single individual. Create your mastermind group. Success will ensue.

"Surround yourself with only people who are going to lift you higher."

-Oprah Winfrey

You are not alone

It is easy to feel isolated while in the company of hundreds of people. But I believe that no matter what it is that is troubling you, there is someone who is either going through the same thing or who understands. Developing friendships in nursing school is important to combat this feeling of isolation and to help you understand that you are not alone.

Understandably, there are people who feel like they just want to stay focused and get through their nursing program unscathed. So, making friends is not on the list of priorities. I am simply suggesting keeping an open mind about it and not take it off the list.

Some instructors will create scenarios where you come out with a friend naturally. Sometimes it is a group project. I know a lot of people hate them, but they aren't all bad. Occasionally being forced to work with someone is what is needed to create a bond. It might be a seat you gravitate to every time you are in a specific class that leads you to be next to a potential friend. You simply need to pay attention and not fight it when the bond begins to form.

Another way to make friends is participating in a study group. Study groups do form in nursing school, but they can be a bit taboo. Consider that because it is not easy to qualify for nursing school, that most students are the "pick of the litter." This means that you may encounter some *strong* personalities and unwavering leadership clashes. Proceed with caution. Even with that, or if you are lucky enough to find a civil and productive study group, it is a place where you may come out with a friend.

The most important thing is that you are open to finding friends. You should not isolate yourself. Neither nursing school nor the profession is a place to be a loner. It is nearly a requirement to have friends or associates. When you have people's lives in your hands and life or death can be solely based off a decision you make, you need someone you can trust and feel comfortable with asking for help.

Friends for life

It is common to stay friends with people you befriended in nursing school. You will connect with the people who you grind out assignments with, celebrate with, laugh with, cry with… these are bonds that will often last a lifetime. These shared emotions are what lasting friendships are built on.

There are nursing students who end up at their first job together, get married, and follow each other through to elevated career goals. It is like personal networking for life partners. These relationships can help you achieve things that may not seem possible. Having someone believe in you from a perspective of an experience that you have lived through together creates trust and understanding that cannot come from other places in your life.

Before nursing school, I was a different person. I considered myself social. I had a group of friends with whom I hung out with occasionally, but I spent most of my free time with family. Once I got accepted into nursing school, this changed for me. Because I went back to college as a nontraditional student and had children, I was past the "let's be friends and hang out" phase that some people go through. I looked at it as a mission. I had never used or joined a study group previously, so it was esoteric to me. It was the furthest from my mind or goals. I ended up befriending a woman who had a very different personality than most of the friends and family who I spent time with. She was energetic (hyper), eloquent, and super smart. I considered myself smart, as well, but it was one of my personality traits that you'd learn once you got to know me on a personal level. We ended up being the only "group" that each of us used to study and for support. We are around the same age, but she had a wealth of wisdom that seemed well beyond her years. Her ability to give and detail scenarios and advice was impeccable—it seemed scripted. She made my experience more tolerable and I learned a lot of life lessons from her. We remained friends from then on. And at the time of this book, 14 years later, we are still friends. She is the only person from nursing school I remained in contact with.

Overall, be sure to have fun. Remember that fun is a collaborative activity. It is also important. Of course, people can have fun alone but most often it is had as a duo or a group of people. Make having fun a priority. Look forward to it. Take pictures. Laugh at yourself. Tell a funny story about class or clinical and laugh together. Take time to create fun memories in the same way that those difficult memories are built.

Try it

Think about all your current close friends. Think back to how and where you met. Answer the following:

1. Did you become friends through a mutually known person? Who was that?
2. Was there an experience you shared that was memorable and bonded you?
3. Did you have a specific conversation? Was there a dialogue? A single but memorable statement? What was it?
4. Was your first encounter none of the above and something completely different? What was that story?

Take time to consider all these questions. I am sure you will find a funny, sweet, or epic story in recalling how you met some or one of your closest friends. It will likely be a lived experience that you shared something fun or life-changing. If you are the sentimental type, write them down and share them with your friend as a gift of your legacy.

Notes

Chapter 7

MENTORSHIP

"Mentoring is a brain to pick, an ear to listen and a push in the right directions."

John C. Crosby

What is a Mentor

As adults, we make choices for different reasons. Sometimes it is directed by the authority figures in our lives, other times choices are self-directed. In either case, when we are serious about learning something new it is not uncommon to seek out someone to help us through the learning process. In this, we look for people who have gone through the path that we are on to give us jewels of wisdom from their mistakes and successes on their journey. When we find such a person we look to them to decrease our anxiety, answer our questions, and give us guidance. This is a mentor.

Benefits

Using a mentor helps you get through some difficult things without the added mistakes that make progress more difficult. You learn from a person who has made all the mistakes that you can now avoid. Many successful leaders had mentors and swear by them. Oprah Winfrey was mentored by Maya Angelou. Bill Gates was mentored by Warren Buffett. Mark Zuckerberg was mentored by Steve Jobs.

Mentors provide advice that comes from a truthful perspective. A mentor does not receive any personal gain by assisting you. They can help you when you are stuck and need to make a difficult decision.

They have connections that you don't have access to. This can increase your level of success by getting you to open doors that you did not know existed. Therefore, they are also an amazing resource for networking.

Studies show that mentorship increases the mentee's chances of success. It enhances leadership—mentors already have the solutions to the problems you are faced with and have the answers you are looking for. They've "been there, done that."

How-To

Make a connection. Pay attention. Ask for some time. Don't be embarrassed or upset if you are turned down. Sometimes people, especially nurses, are very busy. If you are afraid that this may be the outcome, ask in a way that it won't appear to be something overwhelming to your chosen mentor. "Is it okay if I: Arrange a ten-minute phone call a week? Send you an email? Text you a question?" Whatever you must do to make this connection, do not give up.

"Mentoring can also have profoundly positive effects on nursing students and licensed nurses when a good 'match' is made and when mutual interest, respect, and trust are at the center of the relationship."

-Stephanie Wroten & Dr. Roberta Waite. A Call to Action: Mentoring Within the Nursing Profession- *A Wonderful Gift to Give*

Some schools have a structured mentoring program. This points to the fact that there is enough research and understanding for the significance of an importance of mentorship.

Explain yourself. Pitch your plan. People are honored to be asked. You must also understand that you also bring value to your mentor. It is like good parenting. Once people have children, their behavior changes because they want to have a positive impact on their children. Attentive parents know they lead by example. This is the value you add to a mentor. You help them think about their actions and behaviors because they have someone who is following in their footsteps. People who agree to be mentors also like to see their mentees succeed because they have a sense of accomplishment when they assist them in reaching their goals.

You can also have mentors who are no longer alive. How so? As Wil Smith stated, we have access to mentors who have passed on by reading about them in books. Do your research. Look for stories that encompass the inspiring paths of people who did what you are trying to do and overcame significant adversities, and those who had paths similar to your own. And read about those who made it to their goals. This won't have to include historical nurses. It could be anyone with whom you can relate in some way or another because of where they grew up, having some of the same deficits, struggles, family issues, etc.

Become a Mentor

Remember who you were before you got where you are. You can be a mentor right now. Mentor those who are trying to get where you are. Continue to mentor as you are moving through all your milestones. Mentoring makes you a better professional.

I have mentored many people during my time as a nurse and educator. Sometimes it was a formal mentorship, other times it was through me being a trusted colleague and friend. I assisted lots of people through difficult decisions as well as navigating through programs. I feel like it is my duty to "give back" to those who need help in the same way I received help along my journey.

Try it

Think of all the people in your life. Now think of someone you know who is at a perceived level of success, according to you. It does not have to be a nurse. But it should be someone you look up to in some way or another. They may be a parent who seems to keep things together with their children, a leader in the business world, or even a very good student.

1. Come up with some questions you would like to ask them about those things you see them succeeding at and how they relate to your current path.
2. Invite them for coffee, lunch, or dinner. If they are too busy, then ask them if they will give you some time to talk over the phone.
3. In that conversation, ask the questions you came up with.
4. Thank them for taking the time to talk. This is the most important part.

Once you have this activity complete, think about how having answers to some important questions you had gave you a sense of ease. Just the act of getting some things answered by a reliable and respected source can make a big difference in your view. I will bet that this person would be happy that you felt they could help you and that they would check in on you from time to time to see if their advice helped. They would also be more likely to meet with and talk to you again.

Notes

Chapter 8

CLINICAL

Description

Almost all training in the health professions has a clinical portion. It is where the hands-on skills of the profession are learned. This is where students perform in a REAL healthcare setting. Prior to going to clinical, skills are learned in the lab and students must pass a skills assessment to be allowed to practice in the clinical setting. So there are no worries about expecting to perform safely for the first time on patients.

Clinical sites are contracted with the school. All the logistics, rules, and guidelines are spelled out with a school way before students are assigned and show up. Students are prepped on these rules and guidelines by their clinical instructor prior to their first clinical day. On this first day, students learn the ins and outs, locations, get IDs, learn where to park, and things like this.

There are nursing schools that have all "day" clinical rotations. Some others have day, evening, and night rotations. Clinical can be assigned for every day of the week. However, not all schools have weekend rotations. The times range from 6-12 hours. There are generally a wide variety of locations where the students can be assigned. Above all, students do not get to choose their location, day, or time. There are some instances where students can sign up for the evening and night rotations but, in general, the day and time are chosen without input from the students. Why? Because there is not enough time and manpower to do so. The student population will always far outweigh the faculty and staff. It will take too much time to complete and it won't eradicate all the issues that students will come up with for their clinical issues.

Be prepared to adjust to getting up super early in the morning, traveling, and learning the significance of carpooling. As explained above, you may need to adjust to staying up late, as well. Keep an open mind about it because change is inevitable. That is the nature of this profession. If you realize and accept it, the change won't be as painful. You might also learn something new about yourself. If you can't deal with the changes, remember that you can always go back to your routine once you are finished with school.

As a student, one must learn to prepare and be successful in clinical. Clinical information is provided before the first clinical day. Take time out to read it, learn what you need to do beforehand and ask all the important questions before the first day. You don't know what the clinical instructor will be like. There is a chance that he/she will be rigid and strict or laid back. Being prepared will decrease the likelihood of having a negative interaction with either type.

Gather all the supplies needed. Purchase and prepare uniforms. Learn what shoes are appropriate. Socks, underwear, and even the appropriate jackets to be worn. It sounds crazy but students have been sent home for wearing colorful socks and having visible underwear. As far as the jacket is concerned, it gets very cold in hospitals, clinics, and schools, but some places ban sweatshirts and hoodies. So, if you want to bring a jacket with you be sure there are no rules against the one you want to wear. The goal is to look as professional as possible, to represent the school well, and to be as ready for whatever comes that day.

Above all, "walk the line." Learn the rules and follow them. If you make a mistake, own it, learn from it. Unless there is an injustice or something unethical being forced on you, don't make yourself stand out as the person who always has an issue with the rules. Some rules are made from a significant history behind them. Before you feel like you should challenge it, at least learn the history first.

Significance

It is my personal opinion that clinical is the most important part of nursing school. It is where the "rubber meets the road." It is where you get to learn what this "nursing life" is really about. I have known more than one student who completely changed their minds about nursing because of their clinical rotation and left nursing school to never look back. This is not to put a negative spin on it. It is me being honest. Some people don't learn that they despise their chosen profession until they graduate college and get the job that their degree qualifies them for. My son is one of them. Clinical in nursing school affords the benefit of learning this beforehand.

Don't be fooled into thinking that because clinical is pass or fail that this diminishes its significance. A 4.0 "A+" student can still fail because of clinical. If the student cannot perform nursing tasks in a safe and efficient manner they cannot and should not pass. Clinical performance is of major significance. Take it seriously, no matter what!

Taking care of people who need medical care can be difficult. People are vulnerable. Think of yourself and where your confidence lies. It is under a layer of well-done hair, possibly makeup, nice clothing or clothing in general, the shoes of your choice and much more. All that encompasses your identity. Comfort, classy, sophisticated, or stylish. It is part of you. Imagine you are suddenly ill and all the above is taken away. You are then given a gown that barely covers your butt. You suddenly lose all that is who you are in a single bound. Someone who runs a house full of people now needs to ask for assistance to use the bathroom. Imagine the vulnerability. Remember that when you feel like a patient isn't nice. There are layers of things that led up to their behavior. Or it is just who they are. Don't take it personally and don't allow it to keep you from your mission. You are there to learn and find your groove. Keep your eye on the prize.

Other nurses aren't always nice, either, which is another thing to—as best you can—not take personally. I wish this part was one I could leave out of this book. But I would be remiss. Nursing is a tough job. Not everyone can perform it and be nice to nursing students at the same time. Unless there is a personal attack on you, let it go and remember the lesson in it; don't become that nurse to future students who you may encounter.

Make the Best of it

Clinical rotations can be an awesome experience. It is sometimes where students find themselves and feel that they can and will make a difference. So put your best foot forward, wear your best smile, and bring the best attitude.

I always gave my students this advice about clinical:

> "Treat this like a job interview every time you come. Like an athlete playing in front of a scout. Try to stand out. Don't hide

or go get tucked away in a corner on your phone. Most students stand out. Some for the good, others for the bad. When you stand out you will be remembered. Don't believe that you all blend in because you have the same uniforms on. People remember those who make an impact or impression."

I've known more than one student and a family member who stood out for the good and got hired for their performance during clinical. I once had a student who I will never forget because he got offered a job on his first clinical day in his first clinical rotation. He had a very high energetic personality. He was friendly to the staff, visitors, and—most of all—the patients. He was promptly answering all the patient calls. He assisted anyone and everyone he could. Including those not assigned to him or the other students. The nurse manager approached me and asked "who is he? I want to hire him." Unfortunately, he was in a rigorous program and was unable to take the position, but imagine the boost to his confidence.

Make the best of your time in your clinical rotations. Seek out opportunities to perform a task or skill. Ask to watch something being done. Soak it up as much as you can. This is the best time to do it. While you have a clinical instructor at arm's reach who is there for you. Once you graduate there will be a time to learn and develop skills but you will be viewed differently if you don't have the basic skills needed to perform as a new nurse. Remember that the goal is to be safe. One cannot be safe if they have never tried. So get your hands dirty as much as possible. It is the best way to become comfortable with your craft.

Try it

Think of a task that you are currently capable of doing. It could be anything from writing a letter to painting a room. Choose your task. Think of all the things you will need to complete it from start to finish. Make a checklist like this:

1. I will gain or learn_____from this task.
2. Specific attire for the task is _____.
3. The major supplies I will need to complete this are (make a list).

4. These are the rules or special instructions that I need to follow (make another list).
5. I can ask_____to help me.
6. If I run into trouble, I can call _____.
7. It will take me approximately__to finish.
8. When I am finished, I will give it to_____, share it with _____, or take a picture and post it on social media.

This can help you develop the understanding of why clinical rotations are structured the way they are. They are for you to learn. Your attire is to make you look like a professional and to keep your everyday clothing from getting soiled. Also, uniforms make you look uniform. To perform your duties and be prepared to learn, you must have the tools to do so. Nursing is a team and collaborative effort, so most things are done with another person. You must be able to troubleshoot and know the best person to call when you need help. Time management is extremely important. This doesn't mean that you have to rush to do certain things, but if you don't consider time, you will run behind. When you are done, you should view your work with a level of pride or at least completion. If you are not proud, think of how you would do things differently next time and what about this would have made you proud.

Notes

Chapter 9

NETWORKING POWER

"Respect for people is the cornerstone of communication and networking."

-Susan Roane

Six degrees of separation

In theory, everyone in the world is separated by just six people. That means that there are only six people between you and Beyonce', Oprah Winfrey, and Bill Gates… you get what I'm saying. On a smaller scale, there are few people between you and your new position as a graduate nurse. This is, by the way, the goal of completing your program. That said, be mindful of the people you meet and the impressions that you leave on EVERYONE. No one is insignificant. Treat everyone with respect and command it for yourself. You never know who they know and what they will say about you to important people who could impact your future.

It's who you know

Contrary to what you may think and assume by evaluating the number of people around you, the nursing community is small. When there are a lot of people condensed into a small space, you will get an unrealistic sense of the actual population. Everyone knows someone! Understanding this has significant benefits. Networking is powerful in nursing and it starts the first day of nursing school.

If you sit quietly in the corner in every class because you don't want to draw attention to yourself, you are making a huge mistake. This does not translate that being loud and chatty is the best way to be. No, it means that you will go unnoticed. This will not work in your favor when you need a reference from the only people who can vouch for your personality and level of professionalism. It will also not work in your favor when you are struggling or, by some unfortunate circumstance, end up in a situation that you need some help from one of your professors as a person on "the inside."

Talk to people. Meet with your professors. Even if you make up a reason to meet with them. Allow them to get to know you on a personal level.

Not too personal, please. But you understand the gist. Find ways to tell your story of how you got there. What your ultimate goals are. Ask for tips and advice. Get the scoop! Give them a reason to give it to you. "It is the squeaky wheel that gets the oil."

But I digress. Get to know people. Everyone. Not just professors, clinical instructors, and nursing administrators. No one is exempt from who they could potentially reach and connect you to your first and, potentially, dream job. Everyone knows someone who knows someone.

Taking the time to write a *thank you* note or email is also a good way to make an impression and have yourself at the forefront of someone's mind. I am not suggesting that you write random notes to everyone or "kiss up." If someone did something nice, helped you through something difficult, took out their personal time to meet up with you… Take time to thank them. It is the right thing to do. Gratitude will take you further than you can fathom. Expressing gratitude is invaluable. Everyone appreciates being told they are appreciated.

> "Appreciation is a wonderful thing; it makes what is excellent in others belong to us as well."
>
> -Voltaire

Story Time

I went back to nursing school in my late 20s after my children were born. I went in with a background in healthcare. I had a technical career. Therefore, a lot of the initial information in my foundational classes was very familiar to me. I breezed through the classes. At the time, unbeknownst to me, there were some internal scholarships and research studies that had funding allocated to the school I attended. The administrators were "watching" potentially qualified students for this funding. The criteria were that the students had to have an academic record that was in good standing and have good interpersonal skills. So, in other words, you had to stand out from the crowd in your actions and you had to have good grades to match.

Because I had experience with working with the public and most often people who were sick, I understood that it was best that I kept a positive attitude and made a point to be nice. I carried this into nursing school. It was this behavior that got the attention of those making decisions about the previously stated opportunities.

What this got me was more than I could have ever imagined, and I remain grateful. I was given the opportunity to receive money to take other classes in nursing at higher levels than I was currently at. I was in an associate's degree program. Being qualified to participate in this program gifted me with a nursing class on the bachelor's level and the master's level at a well-known university—FREE OF CHARGE. Participating in this initial program granted me the ability to compete for another program that would pay for an internship upon graduation that would not only give me a monthly stipend of $500 but it would also pay for me to go back to the above-noted university to get a bachelor's degree at no cost to me at all. I was selected, and I completed that degree with honors.

At the time that I was completing this internship, I was working full-time as a new nurse. As I think back, I don't know how I did it all. When I graduated from the bachelor's degree program, having one master's level class under my belt, I applied for a graduate degree in nursing. My employee benefits included 100% tuition for two classes per semester. You only needed to pass those classes with a C or better. I went straight back to school to get the degree. I paid for none of it. NONE!

A side note is that I was working for an employer that came to the school I was attending to offer jobs to the seniors. The said school had a great reputation for putting out *the best* nurses in the country. They had received the Centers for Excellence in Nursing Education award more than once. Therefore, the hospitals in the city were known to hire this school's nurse graduates on the spot. My future first nursing employer came to the school and gave a presentation offering a sign-on bonus of

$10,000 to nursing students who agreed to work for them for two years. There were many skeptics who had good explanations for why they would be cautious, but I went with my gut and signed. It was one of the best decisions I ever made, even outside the fact that the $10k was the biggest check made out to me that I had ever seen. To date, this hospital and health system is one of the best known.

All the above is a demonstration of networking and of getting to know people, and how much power it has. I never had a goal of going back to school. I simply wanted to be a nurse. But the stars aligned, and I ended up where I was supposed to be in life. At the completion of the master's program, I was invited to come work for the school where I initially started. It was absolutely amazing. Fast forward to today and I continue to use my networking super-power: I am a professor at a well-known university; A job that I never fathomed I could get as I set my sights on going back to school in my late 20s.

Don't burn bridges

Dare I say it? I will. It does not matter how terrible an instructor, professor, administrator, counselor, classmate… whoever is. It does not matter if you share this feeling about them with 99% of the people in your class. DO NOT ever get comfortable with attempts to "tear them down" for whatever reason you think you should. You never, ever, know who they know, the depth of their reach, and the doors you could potentially close for yourself. Permanently. This is the worst way to start off your nursing career.

One of my colleagues was teaching a group of students who were displeased with one of their other professors. They felt like she was a likely candidate for them (a group) to vent their frustrations to. There was nothing alarming or concerning about their gripes – they simply felt the other professor was not a good instructor. My colleague let them all, one-by-one, express their disapproval of the other professor. She asked them if they expressed their concerns to the professor. They had not. She then turned and called this professor on the phone, while the students were all still in the room. She told the professor that she had a group of students in her presence and detailed out the complaints. There were plenty of red cheeks and looks of surprise in the room. She hung up the phone and turned to them to give them a lesson of being careful of who they vent to about things that could be damaging to someone's career or reputation. That they never know who knows whom and how it can backfire. Have an issue with someone? Tell them first. If you can't or won't tell, then why say anything at all? How does it help anyone?

Of course, you should ABSOLUTELY stand up and advocate for yourself if you need to. But be sure, however, that if you need to handle a situation that involves reporting someone and potentially putting their job on the line, that you handle it with integrity. Handle it in a way that you would hope that if you were in their shoes you would feel you are being treated fairly. Dale Carnegie stated, "Criticism does not produce good or positive outcomes."

If you don't feel like anyone you encounter in your program deserves a compliment and therefore have never given one, you should not feel that is productive or beneficial to be critical and report ANYONE. Understand that a single praise to an instructor, classmate, nurse, professor, or anyone would do more good than a long report would to criticize them. As humans, we are way too quick to point out the bad and not consider the good. Knowing how hard it is to get accepted into nursing school means you know that becoming a nurse, instructor, or professor is a process that is tenfold more difficult. Respect the road they have traveled to be in front of you and seek to understand them before you take the things they say and do personally. If you don't feel comfortable enough to approach them with your concerns, your issue may not be valid.

"Once I did bad... that I heard ever. Twice I did good... that I heard never."

Having enough confidence to approach a person to address an uncomfortable issue will most definitely build character and courage. It will also give the person you have approached a sense of respect for having the esteem and dignity to start with them as the first step to resolve the conflict. Always go the source first. It can be intimidating to do so in the beginning, but once you do it and get past it, it will get less and less difficult. It builds character and leadership skills. Valuable attributes to a nurse or any professional.

Try it

By the time you are at the age to be in nursing school, you could have had many (or at least one) uncomfortable encounter where you were put in a position to explain why you did something. Be it to your parent(s) for something you needed to explain your way out of, in school, work, wherever… think back to the most significant incident. Most notably, an incident where someone else put you in this predicament by reporting or "telling" on you. Recall how it made you feel. Answer the following:

1. Which emotions did you feel about it at the time? Were you angry, anxious, scared, humiliated, or simply upset?
2. How long did the uncomfortable emotions last? Days, weeks, months?
3. When you think about the incident, do the emotions you felt at the time resurface?
4. Did you feel that you were treated fairly?
5. Did this change your relationship with anyone? Did it change your perception of a specific place or thing?
6. Did you learn from it? Did it change you? For the good?

Remember that we are all human. We make mistakes. How mistakes are handled can have positive or negative outcomes for those involved. A misunderstanding or something that can be handled in a face to face conversation can be the best learning tool for all involved, if handled with care.

This activity can have two significant benefits. It will make you more careful when and if you are faced with handling a situation that you need to resolve. It is also therapeutic if you write out the answers to the questions above. Activities, where you write out emotional responses to an experience, can help you get past them.

Notes

Chapter 10

THE NEXT PHASE

"To *begin with the end in mind* means to start with a clear understanding of your destination. It means to *know where you are going* so that you better understand where you are now and so that *the steps you take are always in the right direction.*"

-Dr. Stephen Covey; The 7 Habits of Highly Effective People

This is only the beginning

Getting accepted and getting through nursing school is no small feat. You will feel like you can't wait to get through to the end on almost a regular basis. This is normal and expected. Once you are done, you should be feeling extremely proud of yourself. You have done something amazing and should be celebrated.

As high as you are vibrating after finishing nursing school, as accomplished as you feel, and as relieved as you are to be done… IT IS ONLY THE BEGINNING! You are not finished with learning. The learning curve has merely shifted. You have transformed from the nursing student to the novice nurse. You will feel like you are back at square one. This is ALSO normal and expected. It is one of those things that go along with any new job in any field. However, with more skilled professions, it takes a lot more time to feel confident in your abilities.

The journey

The ultimate goal of completing nursing school is to get a job as a nurse. This may seem simple and easy being that it is widely known and discussed that there is a shortage of nurses. However, getting through the door is not as easy as one may think. Especially as a new grad. Most open positions will be posted for experienced nurses. This is where that networking and getting to know people along the way becomes important.

Those relationships that you built during your time along the way will become your best tool to get to meet your potential new employer. You will need to become a master of networking and creativity by standing out from the crowd of new grads. Sitting in front of the computer and having a "power session" of putting in applications to all the open positions you can find is not the best way to get in the door. This will make you no different than a number. This does not mean that you will NEVER get a job this way, but it is not the most effective method of landing a job as a new nurse.

One of the best ways is to utilize the PEOPLE you have made connections with. Talk to them. Ask if they know anyone you can talk to and reach out to.

Resume

Take the time to craft out a unique and attention-grabbing resume. Make it pleasing to the eye. Some feel like it is acceptable to put pictures and add color to it. Make the information meaningful and stand out. It is not good to have ALL the jobs you held on your resume when you are seeking a new job as a nurse. If you are adding things that are not nursing related, be sure that you tie the job to something of a human connection. For instance, if you worked in retail, be sure to note that you have experience with working with and serving people.

Letters

Writing cover letters are a lost art. Not many people use them anymore unless an application asks for one. However, there is value in a good letter, in general. Not just for job seeking. With a cover letter, be sure to do research for each individual institution that you are looking to apply to. Try to steer clear of generalized cover letters. Take the time to write one for each position. Let the letter speak to how you will fit in the position based off what you have learned in school, what you have researched about the institution, and what you bring to the table, expressed in your personal style.

Never underestimate how you could benefit an institution because you are confident that you are a great person. You know you better than anyone. Think about your positive personality characteristics. Don't be afraid to use them to your advantage. Sell yourself as a great asset to any institution that could have you by explaining what you have to offer. Getting a good job is not just about finding one that will earn you money. It is about a relationship. With all relationships, there is give and take.

You need to think in terms of what you can give to a potential position as well as what a position can give to you. Take this approach once you have been granted an interview.

When selling yourself, be authentic. Don't try to put on a performance that paints a picture of you that is not truthful simply because you want to land the job. Your plan to function as a nurse should be set the day you decide to become a nurse and begin to materialize once you start nursing school. Marketing yourself should be based on the journey that began on day one. Not everyone will have a lively and compelling story, but everyone has a story nonetheless. Sell your story. Sell your services. Tell the facility why they would benefit by having you.

Job fairs

Be on the lookout for job fairs. This is another lost art in nursing. It is more because of a poor understanding of what a job fair is. If an institution takes the time to plan and prepare to have a booth/table at a job fair, there is a chance that there is a great need to fill more than one position. This is another time that you should do some research. Find out what facilities are going to be there. Research each facility's intended qualifications for the positions they are looking to fill. Learn about the mission and vision of the facilities you would like to apply to. Prepare for the event as you would for a job interview. Create neatly packaged documents to give out. Make them individualized, if your research warrants it. Go to the event and give your best! Network, talk to people, and do the on-the-spot interviews. Make it work even if you leave without a prospect, leave an impression.

Stay Positive

During your preparation to seek and secure a job, it is important to remain positive and look at all the good in the experience. Take it all in. Learn as you go. Take notes of the things you are being asked. Look for themes in the questions you note from all the interviewers. Use it to become better at answering them. Take note of each facility that you visit during the interviews. Pay attention to the energy in the space and to the energy coming from those you encounter there. Visualize yourself there as an employee. Note how that visualization makes you feel. Emotional energy is more powerful than you know. By remaining positive and viewing this process as a learning experience, you will be able to tune into your emotions and pay attention to how each person, building, location, conversation, and space makes you feel. Making these connections are also very powerful.

Don't allow yourself to start looking at not being called back as rejection. Allowing negativity to consume you during this process will set you back. This negativity will show up in you during the interviews and conversations, thus pushing you further away from landing a position. You will begin to look, sound, and appear doubtful. Some of your friends and classmates may land jobs almost immediately after graduation, but this does not mean that you are unwanted. It means your journey is different than theirs.

> "May your choices reflect your hopes. Not your fears."
>
> -Nelson Mandela

Try it

If someone asks you "tell me about yourself," you should be prepared to give a brief and compelling description to answer this basic interview question. Many people find this question difficult to answer. The act of selling ourselves by being asked who we are is unusual. Especially being asked this by a stranger. If we are asked more specific questions—such as our favorite television show, food, color or sports team, for instance—we find it easier to answer. Use this as a practice for both a verbal and written response to explain who you are:

1. Tell something about your past:

    - Make sure it is relevant.
    - Where did you grow up?
    - What are your interests, schools, etc.

2. Tell something about yourself presently:

    - What school you graduated from.

- What some of your short-term goals are.
- Any hobbies.

3. Tell something about your future:

   - Where you see your career in the next 5 years.
   - Any significant plans.
   - Going back to school, relocating, entrepreneurship, etc.

If this is a written response, be sure to include how you and your career plans fit into the facility-in-question's mission and vision. Many organization looks for this alignment in prospective candidates. The act of writing it down will also help you remember it when you are asked in a verbal conversation. It will help you with appearing like you know what you want and where you are going.

Notes

Chapter 11

CLOSING

Growing Up

Growing up, I did not know any nurses personally. In fact, most of the health care providers who I remember did not look like me or anyone I knew. Because of this, I never considered that I could be a nurse. One of my aunts and one of my close friend's mother were Licensed Practical Nurses (LPN). Even that seemed too hard to achieve for me. As a young child, this seemed like something you had to have both have money and intelligence to accomplish. Therefore, being a nurse was never anything that I aspired to.

One of the things that helped shape my affinity to health care was how well I did in biology in high school. Biology is the foundation for health sciences. Doing well in this helped me with understanding in class during my time in vocational school and later, nursing school.

Nursing School

I went to nursing school in the middle of North Philadelphia. I was still the minority. I was sure that, somehow, the demographics would be different. I thought that the classes would have a lot of minorities. It did not. They were there, but we were still the minority.

The significance of the demographics was that it was intimidating. You must understand that if you have a built-up perception that you don't belong somewhere—because you have *rarely* seen familiar people in that particular setting—that you could have possibly made a mistake. I am sure that some men who go to nursing school feel the same, being that it is a female-dominated profession.

I did well, but I somehow still felt inferior.

Tragedy

Once I was finishing up my last semester in school, I secured a job before I was even finished, received a $10k bonus, and so many potential benefits in my new position. I quit the pieces of jobs I had (I worked as an extern and was also a tutor) to focus on finals and the NCLEX exam. I was so excited about everything. Life was amazing. I made it.

Three weeks into my new, awesome job, my husband—my rock, my supporter—was murdered. Gunned down in the street. My life changed in a single day.

Prior to this tragedy I had a solid family unit, a stable home and was now entering the career of my dreams. I use the analogy of my life being glass and someone came and shattered it. Broke it into a million pieces. Leaving me to carefully, one by one, pick up the pieces, put them back together and continue the best way I could.

It would have been easy—and most would have understood—to have simply crawled into bed and stayed there indefinitely after that horrific day. It is playing out in my head as I type this, and it is still difficult. But what gave me the strength to continue was that my children needed me. That they did not need to lose both parents. So, I put on a brave face for them. I became the hero in this scenario because I gave them hope. I went back to work and continued with school as planned. To my benefit, this was the best means of coping for me.

Continuing Education

I had a full scholarship that I would lose. This scholarship came with a $500 monthly stipend. I could have taken some time to recover and grieve. But I chose to continue my path. It was what I knew he would have wanted me to do. Thinking of what we talked about and continuing what we planned was where I found my ability to cope. It was the best choice I could have made. I believe that things would be different if this had not happened to me. As morbid as that sounds, I believe that my life changed for the better after his death. I stayed in school. I received two more degrees after he left me so tragically. I am not so sure that I would have kept the stellar trends of staying in school if it weren't for my life changing the way it did.

Being a Professor

It was never a plan for me to become a nursing instructor. It was through networking and the opportunities outlined in the "Networking" chapter that led me to be groomed to teach. It was the exposure and experiences that were provided to me in those activities that I learned that I could be more than a "staff" nurse. Of course, there is an idea of what the path of becoming a nursing instructor was for me, but being that before going back, becoming a nurse seemed way out of reach for me. Therefore, becoming an instructor was unfathomable.

I walked that path anyway. I did not see it becoming real, but I went anyway. It became a reality. I was asked to teach before I had finished my master's degree. Once again, I had a teaching position waiting for me before I was qualified for it. It was like a dream. Not only was it a job, but it was also a highly sought-after position that was by referral only and many were in line before me. The feeling I got from this realization is, to date, difficult to put into words.

I eventually ventured into teaching at other schools and universities. I wanted to gain a wealth of experiences while I was young. I wanted to learn what my fit was in academia. I eventually landed a position at a well-known university in Philadelphia. Prior to this, all my teaching positions were part-time. After a few years working there, I was asked if I wanted a full-time position. Once again, I was invited to take a position that was not easy to obtain or qualify for. I accepted and have been a full Assistant Clinical Professor ever since. My path to this position has been an honorable one.

I have many struggles as a professor. Those struggles are things that come with the territory and things that are specific to me. None of them take away the fact that I still love to teach. I love what it does for me as a nurse, as an educator, and as a person.

Beating the Odds

This closing chapter was added to let you know that we all have struggles and triumph. That our struggles don't have to keep us from achieving our dreams or goals. That it is okay to take the "road less traveled." Every single one of us has things we deal with daily, weekly, monthly, and yearly. It is up to us to use them as an excuse or to use them as a tool.

The odds are always against us. Not many have an easy path. Even when someone is claiming that their path is easy, it is likely a façade because they don't want to appear weak. Don't let setbacks set you back. Use them as momentum. If you want it, then claim it. It is already yours.

Resources

As a Man Thinketh

By James Allen

I loved this book. It is small and mighty. It briefly and thoroughly explains how your thoughts influence your life. By changing your thoughts, you change your life.

Think and Grow Rich

By Napoleon Hill

I recommend this book to anyone who wants, needs or has a job. It has so many gems for people who want to understand how to be successful in life. Albeit to simply be happy or to be rich, this book has something in it for everyone.

How to Win Friend and Influence People

By Dale Carnegie

Like Think and Grow Rich, this book is great for anyone who has or is on their way to earning money while dealing with people. This is one of my favorite books on how to handle people and situations involving people. I have it as an audiobook and regularly re-listen to it. One could learn a lot about successful dealings with people.

A Call to Action: Mentoring Within the Nursing Profession- *A Wonderful Gift to Give*

By Stephanie Wroten & Dr. Roberta Waite.

This is an article on mentorship. This is the only article in this book that I wanted and needed to reference. This is because I personally feel that mentorship is pivotal to success. Whether you are a nurse, doctor, teacher, mom… anything of significance or importance; you need a mentor to do it successfully.

The 7 Habits of Highly Effective People

Dr. Stephen R. Covey

I highly recommend this book to anyone who wants to develop good daily habits. I have personally used the principles in this book and can attest to how your life changes based off those things we do every day that ultimately define who we are. If you want to improve your life and productivity, read this!

Made in the USA
Middletown, DE
02 November 2018